FOOD COMBINING

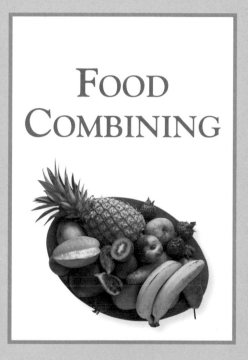

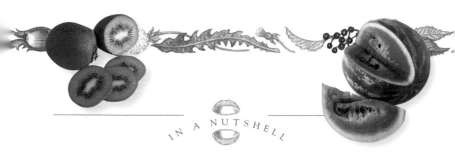

IN A NUTSHELL

FOOD COMBINING
A STEP-BY-STEP GUIDE

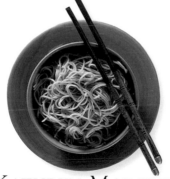

KATHRYN MARSDEN

ELEMENT

SHAFTESBURY, DORSET • BOSTON, MASSACHUSETTS • MELBOURNE, VICTORIA

First published in
Great Britain in 1999 by
ELEMENT BOOKS LIMITED
Shaftesbury, Dorset SP7 8BP

Published in the USA in 1999 by
ELEMENT BOOKS INC
160 North Washington Street,
Boston MA 02114

Published in Australia in 1999 by
ELEMENT BOOKS LIMITED
and distributed by Penguin Australia Ltd
487 Maroondah Highway, Ringwood,
Victoria 3134

NOTE FROM THE PUBLISHER
Unless specified otherwise:
All recipes serve four
All eggs are medium
All herbs are fresh
All spoon measurements are level

Designed and created with
The Bridgewater Book Company Limited

ELEMENT BOOKS LIMITED
Managing Editor Miranda Spicer
Senior Commissioning Editor Caro Ness
Editor Finny Fox-Davies
Group Production Director Clare Armstrong
Production Controller Claire Legg

THE BRIDGEWATER BOOK
COMPANY
Art Director Terry Jeavons
Design and page layout by Axis Design
Editor Jo Wells
Project Editor Caroline Earle
Photography David Jordan
Home Economy Judy Williams
Picture research Caroline Thomas

Printed and bound in Great Britain by
Butler and Tanner Ltd

Library of Congress Cataloging in
Publication data available

ISBN 1 86204 479 1

*The publishers wish to thank the following for
the use of pictures:* Tony Stone Images: 6,
10, 12, 16, 22, 23, 29B, 36. CORBIS/
Bettmann: 8. Image Bank: 20, 21, 28, 45T,
47T. Science Photo Library: 11 (both). A-Z
Botanical: 37.

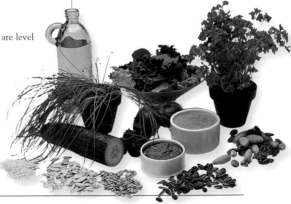

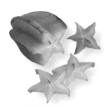

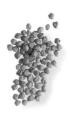

Contents

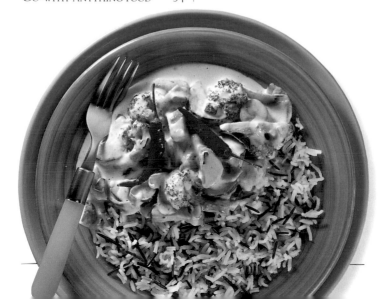

What is food combining?

FOOD COMBINING *follows the simple premise that proteins and starches should not be combined at the same meal: in fact, 'food separation' would perhaps be a better description, as the very word 'combining' conveys mixing things together rather than keeping them apart. For example, the food we call 'high-quality' or 'first class' proteins (principally meat, poultry, fish, soy, eggs, and milk products) do not mix very well with the very starchy foods (bread, potatoes, and cereals).*

The way in which proteins and starches are digested underlies this theory. Proteins are broken down by acid gastric juices in the stomach: almost as soon as a single piece of meat, chicken, or fish has been swallowed, hydrochloric acid is produced.

The digestion of starches is rather different. Bread, potatoes, and cereals begin their digestive journey when they come into contact

BELOW **Mixing "foods that fight" can lead to indigestion.**

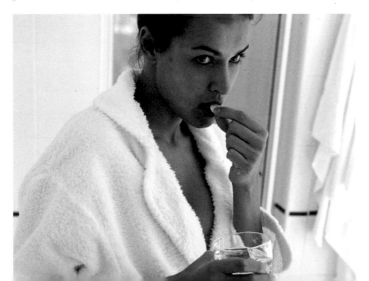

FOODS THAT FIGHT

Proteins

- Meat
- Poultry
- Game
- Fish
- Eggs
- Milk
- Cheese
- Soy

Starches

- Bread
- Cakes
- Cookies
- Wheat
- Oats
- Barley
- Rye
- Bran
- Corn
- Potatoes
- Rice

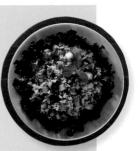

RICE WITH
MINT AND
RAISINS

FISH WITH
TOMATOES
AND OLIVES

with the alkaline juices of the mouth. This process continues in the stomach for 40 to 60 minutes and breaks the starch into smaller components to prepare it for further digestion in the small intestine. As soon as gastric acids are triggered by proteins, the enzymes in saliva are inactivated and starch digestion stops.

If a meal is consumed that contains both starches and proteins, the process of digestion slows right down. Studies suggest that this could be because there is too much acidity to allow the continued digestion of the starch but not enough to break down the protein properly. This can mean that food lingers in the digestive system for too long, encouraging fermentation, a build-up of gas and production of toxins. Some digestion will take place, but it is incomplete.

Proteins and starches are sometimes referred to as **foods that fight.**

A short history

THE FIRST *known use of food combining is attributed to a highly organized religious sect known as the Essenes, who lived in Palestine around 2,000 years ago.*

Dr William Howard Hay developed his own food-combining formula during the 1920s when his health was failing and his medical colleagues could find no treatment to help him. Seriously overweight and suffering from kidney and heart complaints, he turned his attention to nutritional therapy in an effort to resolve his symptoms.

NUTRIENT ABSORPTION

One particular area of research caught his attention. In the mid-1800s, a group of American doctors had discovered that digestion and absorption could be seriously impaired if foods were eaten in the wrong combinations. Further study confirmed that when the body doesn't digest efficiently, the resulting toxicity could cause or aggravate health problems.

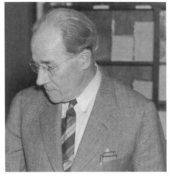

ABOVE **Dr William Howard Hay used food combining to improve his health.**

THE HAY DIET

Dr Hay took these basic principles and used them to develop his own nutrition system. It became known as the Hay Diet. As a result, he was able not only to cure his own ailments and to lose an excess of 56 pounds, but he was also able to use his methods to help many of his patients reclaim their own good health.

DR LUDWIG WALB

In the late 1930s, Dr Hay's success caught the attention of a German physician, Dr Ludwig Walb, who introduced similar food-combining methods to patients at his clinic. He saw significant improvements in a wide range of illnesses—asthma, diabetes, digestive problems, rheumatism and arthritis, kidney disease, and obesity.

DR HERBERT SHELTON

Dr Shelton spent almost 50 years compiling data on how different food combinations affect health. He is still regarded by many practitioners as the guru of food-combining methods.

These are two approaches to food combining: the Hay Diet and a simplified style based on the teachings of Dr Shelton and others. Both work equally well.

FOOD COMBINING

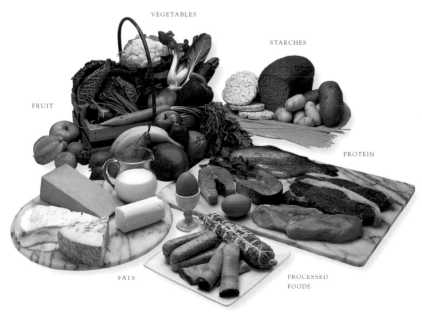

VEGETABLES

STARCHES

FRUIT

PROTEIN

FATS

PROCESSED FOODS

The benefits of food combining

THE FOOD-COMBINING *program is easy to follow, needs no specialty knowledge, and uses everyday foods. This small, but comprehensive guide provides the basic principles for a simple food-combining eating plan.*

Improving diet as a way of improving the quality of life and reducing the risk of illness is gaining far wider acceptance, both medically and scientifically.

But there is more to maintaining optimum health than simply sticking to a high-fiber, low-fat, low-salt diet. Even the most perfectly balanced diet will not be of any value unless the food is properly digested and absorbed by your body. An increasing number of medical practitioners are discovering that food combining can help their patients to improve digestion and absorption of vital nourishment, resulting in an increase in energy levels, balanced body weight, and enhanced general wellbeing.

BELOW *Modern methods produce large quantities of processed foods.*

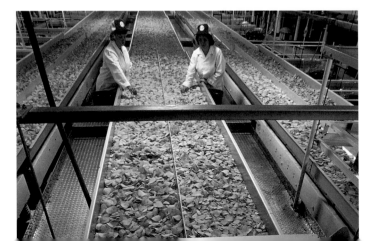

MODERN HEALTH

In the technological world, better hygiene, the benefits of indoor sanitation, and the advent of antibiotics and vaccinations, have all played their part in eradicating infectious diseases, such as diphtheria, smallpox, and tuberculosis. Modern methods of food production, transportation, and storage ensure that most people have enough to eat.

Yet less than perfect health is still a factor in the lives of many. A whole array of insidious and debilitating disorders exists— rheumatoid arthritis, multiple sclerosis, cardiovascular diseases, and cancer. Asthma, allergies, ulcers, irritable bowel syndrome, and chronic fatigue syndrome are all on the increase. Obesity is becoming more common.

No one could doubt the value of modern medical and surgical technology in improving the world's health, but the

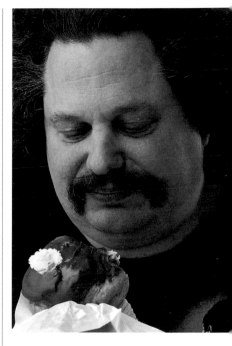

ABOVE *Obesity is an increasingly common health problem.*

realization is dawning that, if one is to make any impact on current statistics, attention must be focused on preventing disease, rather than waiting for it to happen and then taking action.

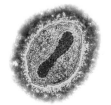

LEFT *Vaccines have helped eradicate viruses such as smallpox.*

HEALTH BENEFITS

Keeping major proteins and starches away from each other allows the body to digest food more efficiently and increases the prospect of better long-term health. Combining foods more carefully may also benefit anyone trying to lose weight.

Those who follow food-combining methods have reported improvements in a whole range of conditions including hay fever and other respiratory allergies, food allergies, arthritis, high cholesterol, recurring and minor infections, migraine, and skin conditions, such as eczema, psoriasis, acne, and urticaria. Heartburn, ulcers, irritable bowel syndrome, constipation, diarrhea, bloating, and flatulence are often considerably relieved—and, in many cases, completely resolved—by the introduction of more careful food combinations.

Food combining increases the efficiency of the digestive system. As a likely result, more nutrients are absorbed—a sound reason not to mix foods that fight.

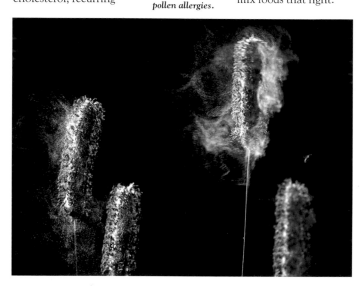

BELOW *Food combining can reduce many ailments including pollen allergies.*

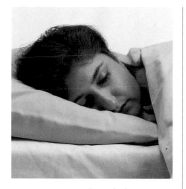

ABOVE *Disturbed*
sleep patterns may
respond well to a
change in diet.

WEIGHT LOSS

In addition, food combining has
proved to be a very successful
route to weight loss, especially if
the usual calorie-counting diets
have not worked or have been
effective only in the short term.

Although food combining
has been shown to be helpful for
so many conditions, it is not a
cure-all. However, anyone who is
plagued by persistent ill-health
or unresolved weight problems,
particularly if they have found
no relief from other types of
treatment, could well benefit
from introducing some food-
combined meals into their
weekly menu.

TARGET AILMENTS AND ILLNESSES

Practitioners, patients, and
food-combining researchers
have found that the following
respond well to food combining.

- Bloating
- Constipation
- Diarrhea
- Flatulence
- Heartburn
- Irritable bowel syndrome
- Ulcers
- High cholesterol
- Palpitations
- Panic attacks
- Acne
- Eczema
- Psoriasis
- Urticaria
- Irritability
- Sleep problems
- Stress
- Allergies
- Arthritis
- Hay fever
- Minor infections
- Lethargy/lack of energy
- Migraine
- Obesity

Science and good sense

DESPITE THE POPULARITY of food combining, it has attracted skepticism from some quarters. There are three main objections. Firstly, that there is insufficient scientific evidence to support the theory that mixing proteins and starches interferes with digestion; secondly, that the body is designed to cope with mixed meals, and thirdly, that most foods contain both protein and starch anyway—so why bother to separate them?

There is, in fact, much evidence to support food combining. Apart from the work carried out by Dr Hay in the 1920s and 1930s, Dr Herbert Shelton carried out food-combining studies from 1930 to 1980. Dr Ludwig Walb studied Dr Hay's work in detail and adopted the Hay Diet as a standard treatment in his clinic.

However, less research has been carried out in recent years and it is still not absolutely certain how and why the system works.

MIXED MEALS
Mixed meals are a relatively modern introduction. Our digestive system has hardly evolved from that of our hunter-gatherer ancestors, who were far more used to eating foods individually than mixed together. They ate meat when they were able to catch it and fruits, roots, nuts, berries, and seeds when available.

It is indeed true that nearly all foods, even vegetables,

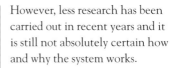

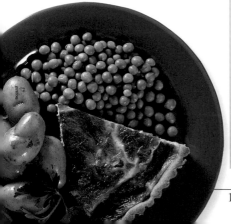

LEFT **A traditional "mixed" meal—peas, quiche, and potatoes.**

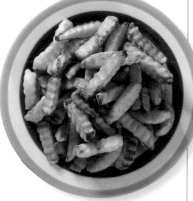

ABOVE *The starch in fries will not be digested fully when eaten with protein.*

protein and ⅟₅₆ ounce of starch, not enough of either to interfere with digestion. The same weight of steak or turkey breast has over ¾ ounce of protein and needs a considerable output of gastric acid to be digested. Fries have about 1 ounce of starch, which will not be digested fully if the stomach is already acid.

The percentage of protein or starch in each food decides its food-combining category.

contain both protein and starch, but when proteins and starches

CAULIFLOWER

occur in foods in only very small amounts, they do not require the same level of digestive effort as the high-quality ones. A 3½-ounce cauliflower floweret, for example, contains ⅟₁₀ ounce of

RIGHT *High-protein foods, such as steak, should be eaten with other proteins, vegetables, or salad.*

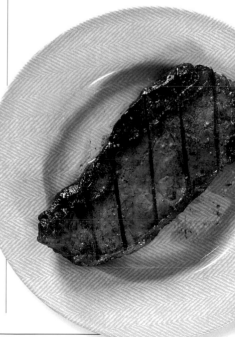

15

Different approaches

IF THERE IS *one main difficulty attached to food combining, it is that there are so many different approaches to the system. An array of healthy eating programs is based to a greater or lesser degree on fundamental food-combining guidelines. There are many which, even though they make no mention of the phrase "food combining," still follow its basic principles.*

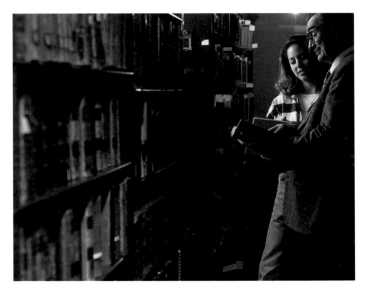

Some approaches are more complicated than others and some are extremely strict. A few suggest standards that, although they may work very effectively in ideal circumstances, completely

ABOVE *The volume of books on this subject can be bewildering.*

fail to make any allowances for our constantly changing and usually hectic lifestyles.

KEEP IT SIMPLE

Anyone who has tried the Hay Diet or another food-combining diet, but gave up because it seemed too complicated, should be inspired to start again. As long as you follow the basic rule of not mixing major proteins with major starches, confusion need not arise.

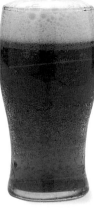

ABOVE *Beer is a starchy food.*

food-combining route. They include experts such as Annemarie Colbin, Wayne Pickering, Luc De Schepper, Dr Jonn Matsen, Doris Grant and Jean Joice, Michel Montignac, and Harvey and Marilyn Diamond. Clinical work has shown that food combining does not have to be complex to be effective.

All types of food combining seem to work well for most people and it certainly is not necessary to eat everything separately or to follow strict food-combining rules at every single meal on every day of the week.

OTHER SUPPORT

Apart from doctors Hay, Shelton, and Walb, a number of other leading nutritional and medical writers have followed the

RIGHT *As a general rule, avoid fatty, sugary, and processed foods.*

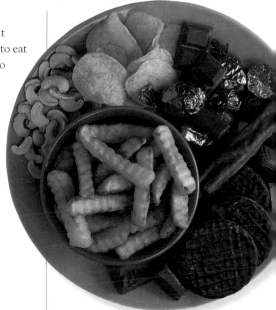

Transit times

TO UNDERSTAND FULLY *the importance of careful food combinations it is necessary to understand that different foods take varying lengths of time to pass through the digestive system.*

M ost of us eat mixed meals —some kind of protein (meat or fish), accompanied by a starchy food (potatoes or rice), and vegetables, followed by fruit or a sweet dessert. We chew and swallow it and expect the digestive system to take what is needed and discard the waste.

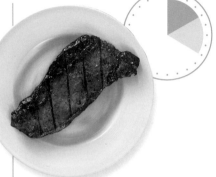

ABOVE *Protein foods need several hours to be digested fully.*

LISTEN TO YOUR BODY

Often the only time we give thought to our bodies is when they cause discomfort.

The length of time that it takes to digest food will vary from person to person, depending on a number of factors—including the general health of the digestive system and how the foods are combined. However, there are certain generalizations that hold true. Most animal-based proteins

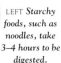

LEFT *Starchy foods, such as noodles, take 3–4 hours to be digested.*

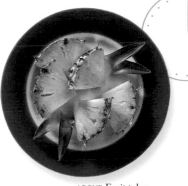

together, it is easy to see how the digestive process not only slows right down, but also becomes inefficient.

ABOVE *Fruit takes 20–40 minutes to be digested.*

take from four to eight hours to be broken down. If digestive capability is poor, some studies suggest 72 hours may be required.

Starchy foods are digested more quickly, in three to four hours; fruit in about half an hour.

INEFFICIENT EATING

When foods that need different transit times and different conditions are chewed up

DESSERTS

Humans have, unfortunately, acquired an unnatural desire to eat something sweet after a main meal. Sugary and refined foods interfere with stomach acid and increase the risk of fermentation. If you cannot cut out sweets, then it can help to leave a gap of an hour between the main course and a dessert.

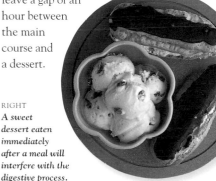

RIGHT
A sweet dessert eaten immediately after a meal will interfere with the digestive process.

RELATIVE TRANSIT TIMES		
Protein	meat, poultry, cheese, fish, eggs	4 to 8+ hours
Starch	potato, bread, rice, pasta	3 to 4 hours
Fruit	from apples to water melon	20 to 40 minutes
Vegetables	from artichokes to zucchini	variable timings

Suitability

FOOD COMBINING *appears to help a considerable number of people suffering from a wide range of health problems. So far, there have been no reports of any adverse reactions or unwanted side effects. However, for medical reasons, there are those who may find a food-combining regime unsuitable.*

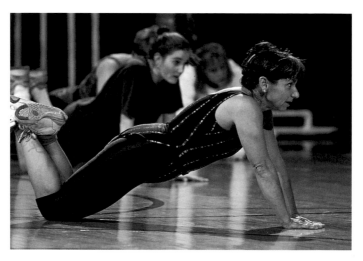

There are reports of fitness teachers recommending food combining to those in their gym and aerobic classes. They say that the diet appears to improve the balance of blood glucose and reduce the risk of hypoglycemic attacks during exercise routines.

ABOVE *Some fitness coaches recommend food combining.*

GRAY AREAS

There are two types of people for whom food combining may not be suitable. Although it is well known for encouraging healthy weight loss, those who are of lean build and hypermetabolic (have a fast metabolism), may find that their metabolic rate slows down a little if they remain on a mixed diet. However, some underweight people fare extremely well. Where low body weight is caused by poor absorption of nutrients, food combining may help to increase weight. People who have lost weight as a result of surgery or illness have also found that food combining helps to restore their weight to normal.

A few articles have been published that suggest food combining may be unsuitable for those with insulin-resistance, a condition in which insulin becomes less effective at controlling blood glucose. Permanently raised glucose levels are associated with diabetes and could increase the risk of cardiovascular disease.

However, food combining has succeeded in improving diabetic control. Dr Hay used the system to treat patients suffering from late-onset non-insulin-dependent diabetes. More recently, a number of diabetics, some treated with insulin, some by diet only, and others on tablet medication, have found food combining helps them to control their condition more efficiently.

CAUTION

Before embarking on any new diet or exercise program, it is important that you consult a medically qualified practitioner to make sure that it will suit you.

This is especially important for anyone who is pregnant, is suffering from any diagnosed medical condition, such as diabetes or allergies, or is taking regular prescribed medication.

RIGHT **Consult your doctor before starting a new dietary regime.**

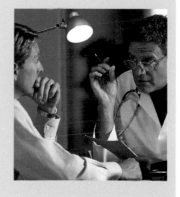

Weight loss

FOOD COMBINING *has long been recognized for its health-promoting benefits. By food combining Dr Hay improved his health and found, almost by accident, that he could shed excess weight. However, it is only in recent years that food combining has gained popularity as a successful method of losing weight.*

Food combining and dieting to lose weight are not the same thing. Diets are usually seen as something to "go on" and "come off," are generally associated with calorie counting, and are based on the premise that to weigh less, you must eat less. But most diets work only while you are "on" them and long-term dieting for weight loss is not healthy.

A DIFFERENT WAY OF THINKING

Food combining goes against current nutritional thinking regarding weight loss. Unlike most diets, it has nothing to do with counting calories, but instead encourages three good meals per day and does not restrict portion sizes.

Researchers have been unable to determine exactly why food combining is so effective at

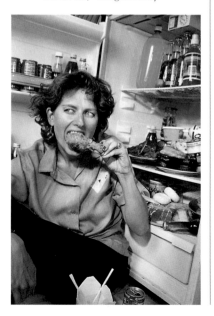

LEFT **Food combining may help to reduce the urge to binge.**

LOSING WEIGHT SUCCESSFULLY WITH FOOD COMBINING

- Forget completely about counting calories
- Follow the two basic rules (see page 26)
- Serve portions that satisfy your appetite, but do not overeat
- Food combine for a few days each week to maintain your target weight
- Exercise regularly

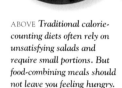

helping to maintain a healthy, stable weight, but there are several theories. Some practitioners have observed that food combining balances blood-sugar levels, reducing the risk of cravings which often result in binges.

Others say that, because digestion is improved, more of the vitamins and minerals needed to burn energy are absorbed. A food-combining approach also

ABOVE *Traditional calorie-counting diets often rely on unsatisfying salads and require small portions. But food-combining meals should not leave you feeling hungry.*

RIGHT *Increased energy levels encourages more exercise and activity.*

often lifts lethargy and increases energy levels, with the result that people feel more inclined to exercise.

A GRADUAL IMPROVEMENT

Weight loss on a food-combining diet is not rapid: expect to lose no more than about 2 pounds a week. But remember that weight lost slowly is less likely to creep back than weight which falls off quickly.

Allergies

FOOD COMBINING *can be of immense value to people who have a limited diet owing to food sensitivity. When we find that certain foods upset us, we may choose to avoid them. If that situation applies to just one or two items, then we should come to no harm. However, if our systems become sensitive to a wider range of foods, the quality and quantity of our intake is affected, increasing the risk of malnourishment and vitamin/mineral deficiency.*

While food allergies have become a health problem in their own right, real allergies are quite rare. More common is food sensitivity or intolerance.

Food combining appears to relieve the symptom of food sensitivity by improving digestive efficiency. Partially digested food provides a cozy

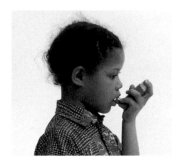

ABOVE **Asthma is increasingly common.**

GLUTEN INTOLERANCE

Suitable starches for someone suffering from gluten intolerance

- rice
- potatoes and parsnip
- buckwheat
- millet
- corn

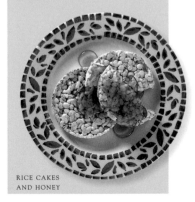

RICE CAKES AND HONEY

environment for unfriendly bacteria which, if allowed to proliferate, can produce toxic substances that are then absorbed into the bloodstream.

THE IMMUNE SYSTEM

If proteins are not broken down fully by stomach acids, they may be absorbed in a more complex form that the immune system does not recognize.

As with any alien substance, the body reacts by trying to eliminate the invader. This could be a major source of immune system stress and allergic reactions. By helping to support the immune system, food combining may also help reduce respiratory allergies.

DIGESTIBLE COMBINATIONS

When assessing the effects of food combining Dr Shelton observed that food allergies cleared up completely when allergic individuals used what he called "digestible combinations." In other words, it was the incompatible combinations of certain foods that were causing symptoms, not the individual

COMMON ALLERGENS

There are a few foods and chemicals which, because they appear to cause reactions in so many people, are worth cutting down or even avoiding altogether. These include:

- beef
- pork
- cow's milk products
- nuts
- peanuts
- artificial flavorings, colorings, and preservatives

CHEESE

- sugar
- processed bread
- wheat
- cereals
- yeast

ARTIFICIAL COLORINGS

PROCESSED BREAD

foods themselves. Today's food-combining practitioners confirm Dr Shelton's findings.

Keep it simple

THE SECRET *of food-combining success is to keep things simple. First familiarize yourself with the two most important rules.*

You can use the basic food-combining principles as the stepping stones to improving your energy levels, digestive function, and overall health and wellbeing. But your everyday life will impose its own constraints. Accept that compromise will be necessary and don't worry if you don't get it right every time.

RULE 1

Eat fruit on an empty stomach. Before you introduce Rule 2, it will help to follow Rule 1, the Fruit Rule, for a full week. That way, you'll be used to eating fruit separately and already helping your digestion to work more efficiently. You should also find that you are eating more fruit than before.

FRUIT AND JUICES

Do eat fruit or drink juices

● First thing in the morning

● Between meals

● As a starter or aperitif

GLASS OF FRUIT JUICE

Don't eat fruit or drink juices

● With other foods

● As a dessert

● In the middle of a meal

BANANAS

LEFT *Adopting a food-combining approach does not mean that you have to give up your favorite foods; enjoy them once in a while.*

RULE 2

Do not combine proteins and starches at the same meal.

To learn which foods combine best, consult the chart on pages 32 and 33.

Rule 2 can be a daunting prospect. It can be difficult to face a diet that says no more pizza, burgers and fries, or pasta and bolognese. But there is no need to avoid these familiar combinations forever. If you have a real craving for a particular protein and starch dish, then allow yourself to enjoy it—perhaps once or twice a week. If you are combining carefully for about five days out

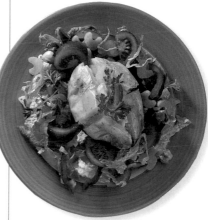

ABOVE *Starches go well with vegetables or salads.*

of seven, or for two meals out of three, then you should still benefit considerably.

BE FLEXIBLE

It is hardly ever possible to eat the perfect diet. Be flexible; do the best that you can. Remember that vegetables and salads can be combined with any kind of protein or starch.

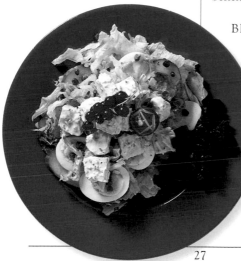

LEFT *Eggs and tofu with salad and beetroot is a good protein and vegetable combination.*

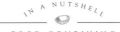
The fruit rule

FRUIT IS AN *important part of any healthy eating plan and is essential for anyone following a food-combined diet. But how and where does it fit into food combining? It is not considered a high-class protein nor is it starchy like bread, pasta, or potatoes. Do we eat it with proteins, with starches, or should it be consumed entirely separately from other foods? Those responsible for early research were not able to agree on this point.*

Dr Shelton's own studies found that fruit does not mix well with other foods. His research confirmed that if fruit is part of a main meal or is eaten as a dessert, it can interfere with digestion.

The majority of practitioners and researchers of modern food combining, including those who followed the Shelton lead, agree that fruit should be eaten separately.

The only anomaly to

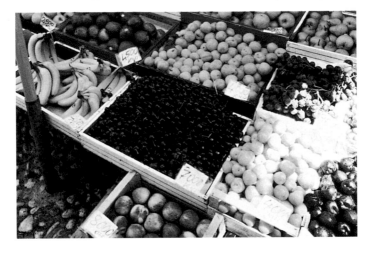

BELOW *An appetizing display of fresh fruit on a market stall.*

isn't clear. Eating fruit with other foods is specific to the Hay philosophy and is still adhered to by those who remain devoted to Dr. Hay's approach. A number of practitioners have reported that keeping fruit entirely separate from other food seems to be especially beneficial to people who suffer from any kind of digestive or bowel disorder—heartburn, stomach ulcers, bloating, flatulence, irritable bowel or malabsorption syndrome.

ABOVE *Fruit and yogurt combine happily.*

this is the combination of fruit and yogurt, which seem to fit comfortably together. This is probably because, unlike other proteins, yogurt is very easily digested.

THE HAY APPROACH

Dr Hay was alone in believing that acid fruit could be eaten with any kind of protein and very sweet fruits with starchy foods. Why Dr Hay was at variance with other opinions

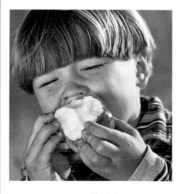

ABOVE *Fruit is a healthy and convenient between-meals snack.*

Eat more fruit

ONE OF *the many benefits of food combining is that it encourages us to eat more fruit and vegetables. But while vegetables are very versatile because they combine with proteins or starches, fruit can create havoc in the digestive system.*

Fruit travels through the digestive system much more quickly than proteins or starches and requires less energy to digest. However, if it is eaten with or immediately after an ordinary meal, it remains in the stomach for too long. Any starches will begin to ferment and proteins to putrefy. This results in a build-up of gas in the digestive system, which, in turn, leads to an increased risk of heartburn, bloating, and flatulence.

A HEALTHY CHOICE?

When people say that they cannot eat fruit because it "disagrees" with them, it could be the combination of fruit with other food, rather than the fruit itself, that is causing the problem. If we choose fruit salad as a dessert, for example, it is often because we think fruit is the healthiest option. Fruit is a healthy choice to make, but it is more likely to be digested easily if eaten separately.

• Eat fresh fruit or drink fruit juice when you first get up in the morning. If you eat breakfast after you've bathed and dressed, the fruit will be well on its way to being properly digested before any other food arrives in your digestive system.

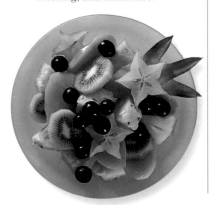

LEFT **Fruit salad makes a revitalizing snack.**

FRUIT SUGGESTIONS

Apples

Bananas

Boysenberries

Breadfruit

Cherries

Dates

Figs

Grapefruit

Hunza apricots

KIWI FRUIT

Kiwi fruit

Lemons

Lychees

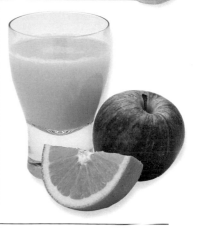

STAR FRUIT

Mandarins

Nectarines

Oranges

Passion fruit

Pears

Pineapples

Red currants

Satsumas

Tangerines

Apricots

Blackberries

Carambola (star fruit)

Durian

Grapes

Limes

Mangoes

Paw-paw (papaya)

Raspberries

Strawberries

Black currants

Clementines

Guavas

Loganberries

Melons

Peaches

Blueberries

Cranberries

MELON

- Eat fruit on an empty stomach either as a between-meals snack or before a main meal.

- Aim for two pieces of fruit and a glass of fresh juice each day. Combine different fruits as fruit salads or juice medleys. Dried fruits are nutritious and make delicious compotes.

RIGHT *Fruit is an excellent way to start the day.*

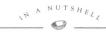

Proteins and starches

AVOID FOODS THAT FIGHT—*that is follow the simple rule of not eating foods that are high in protein with those that are high in starch at the same meal.*

The charts below and opposite list the most common main types of protein foods and starchy foods for easy reference. For example, a meal of chicken and salad or pasta and roast vegetables.

PROTEINS

Protein foods mix well with all kinds of salad foods, any vegetables (apart from potatoes), oils, spreading fats, nuts, and seeds. Proteins do not mix well with starches or fruits.

MAJOR PROTEINS

Meat	Poultry	Dairy products	Soy	Other
Beef	Chicken	Butter	Soy milk	Eggs
Game	Turkey	Milk	Soy products	Myco-
Lamb	Duck	Cheese	Bean curd	protein
Pork		Yogurt	TVP (textured	
			vegetable protein)	

BELOW *Meat, cheese, eggs, and milk are all rich protein sources.*

STARCHES

Starches mix well with any salad foods, vegetables (including potatoes), nuts, seeds, dressings, oils, or spreading fats. Starches do not mix with proteins or fruits.

STARCHY FOODS

Grains	Pasta	Bread	Cereals	Other
Barley	Kamut	Rye bread	Porridge	Potatoes
Buckwheat	Spelt	Soda bread	Muesli	Sweet
(kasha)	Durum	Rice cakes	Corn	potatoes
Oats	semolina	Rye crackers	Couscous	Yams
Quinoa	Buckwheat	Oat crackers	All types	Cake
Brown rice	pasta	Pita	of flour	Sweet
White rice		Ciabatta	Rye	cookies
Basmati rice		Matzos		All types of
Wild rice				lentil, pea,
Semolina				and bean
				except
				soy)

BELOW *Starchy foods, such as bread, grain, cereals, and pasta, tend to be filling.*

Go-with-anything foods

EATING PROTEINS AT *a different meal from starches raises the question "what can we eat with them once they are separated?" One group of foods lends itself brilliantly to the food-combining system— salads and vegetables, labeled here as the "go-with-anything" foods.*

With the exception of potatoes, which are very starchy, vegetables and salads do not contain enough protein or starch to require a special category and will be digested in either an acid or alkaline stomach. Consequently, they can be combined successfully with meat, poultry, fish, cheese, eggs, or soy products on the one hand, or bread, potatoes, and cereals on the other.

Other foods that go with anything are herbs, spices, seeds, nuts, oils, and fats.

Use the chart (opposite page) as a quick check of which foods combine favorably with which. It is good to combine any of the foods in the middle column with either protein or starches, but do not mix the left and right columns together.

NEUTRAL FOODS

Some books refer to some foods as 'neutral' because they are neither mainly protein nor starch. But the word 'neutral' is used to describe pH levels (*see page 42*) so the term 'go-with-anything' is used instead.

LEFT **Broiled chicken breast combined with roasted red bell peppers and salad.**

PROTEINS	GO-WITH-ANYTHING	STARCHES
Fish	All vegetables (except potatoes)	Potatoes
Shellfish		Sweet potatoes
Poultry	All salads	Yams
Bean curd	All types of seeds	Corn
Eggs	Herbs and spices	All types of flour
Meat	Nuts	All grains, including anything made from: barley, buckwheat, couscous, oats, quinoa, rice, rye, semolina.
Milk	Sesame seed paste	
Buttermilk	Pesto	
Cheese	Salad dressings	
Yogurt	Spreading fats, including: butter and margarine	
TVP (textured vegetable protein)	Cooking oils, including: olive oil and sunflower oil	Cereals, muesli, porridge
Soy	Cream	Pasta
		Cookies
		Cake
		Breads, including: rye bread, soda bread, rice cakes, rye crackers, oat crackers, pita, ciabatta, matzos

BELOW *Oils, salads, herbs, nuts, seeds, pesto, and sesame seed paste "go with anything."*

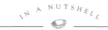
Vegetables

EVERYONE'S DIET SHOULD CONTAIN *plenty of vegetables.*
In terms of food combining, vegetables can be included as part of any
type of meal, whether it is starch or protein.

A diet that contains plenty of vegetables is a healthy one. Vegetables are a good source of fiber, vitamins, and minerals. They also contain a range of phytochemicals, some of which are believed to protect the body and to help it to fight infection and disease. Several studies have shown a link between a diet rich in vegetables and a low risk of cancer.

BELOW *The fresher the vegetables, the more nutritional value they have.*

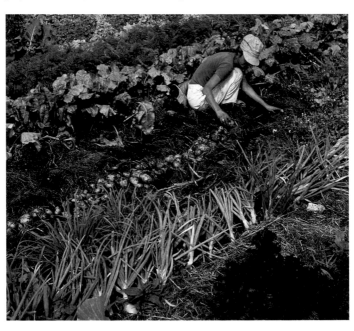

GREEN	ROOT	HERB	OTHER
Asparagus	Beets	Basil	Artichokes
Beet greens	Carrots	Bay	Avocado
Green bell peppers	Celery root	Chervil	Bamboo
Broccoli	Garlic	Chives	shoots
Mustard and cress	Ginger	Dill	Bean sprouts
Snow peas	Onions	Fennel	and other
Spinach	Rutabaga	Marjoram	sprouted
Sugar snap peas	Scallions	Mint	seeds
Turnip greens	Turnips	Parsley	Eggplants
Squash	Fennel	Rosemary	Mushrooms
Watercress		Sage	Tomatoes
Zucchini		Tarragon	
Brussels sprouts		Thyme	
Green cabbage			
Cauliflower			
Collard greens			
Celery			
Belgian endive			
Dandelion greens			
Endive			
Kale			
Lettuce			

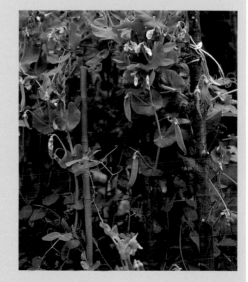

RIGHT *Garden fresh
peas in their pods
are delicious lightly
steamed.*

Pulses

PULSES, OR LEGUMES, *present a thorny contradiction. With the exception of soy, they are "low-quality" or "second class" proteins. However, they also contain significant amounts of starch.*

D r Hay viewed pulses as a troublesome food because they could be difficult to digest and could cause quantities of gas. He recommended they be avoided. But pulses are nutritious and provide an important protein source for vegetarians and vegans.

HEALTH BENEFITS
Research shows that pulses help to lower blood pressure, blood glucose, and cholesterol. They also aid bowel function and may inhibit some types of cancer.

ADUKI BEANS

BLACK BEANS

COMPOSITION
Black-eyed peas, butter, kidney, garbanzo and navy beans, lentils, and most other pulses are made of two-thirds starch and one-third protein.

Peanuts are a pulse and, like soy beans, contain around two-thirds protein and one-third starch. Treat both soy and peanuts as major protein foods and all other pulses as starch. Long green beans have a low starch/protein content and can be treated as "go-with-anything" vegetables.

Sprouted beans are not starchy and are alkaline-forming, "go-with-anything" vegetables.

Snow peas, sugar snap peas, petit pois, and garden peas are classed as vegetables, not pulses.

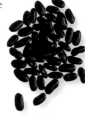

RED
KIDNEY BEANS

AMINO ACIDS
The value of any protein is determined by how many amino

NAVY BEANS

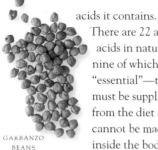

GARBANZO
BEANS

acids it contains. There are 22 amino acids in nature, nine of which are "essential"—they must be supplied from the diet and cannot be made inside the body. To be classed as a high-quality protein, a food must contain these nine essential amino acids. Eggs, meat, poultry, cheese, fish, milk, yogurt, and soy beans fall into this group. Beans other than soy are not complete proteins because they are short of one or more of the nine essential amino acids.

Hummus is made with garbanzo beans, so it does not combine well with protein foods. Instead combine hummus with starchy foods, such as baked potatoes, bread, or crackers.

To reduce the risk of indigestion, cook pulses thoroughly and chew them well.

BELOW *Combine hummus with other starchy foods.*

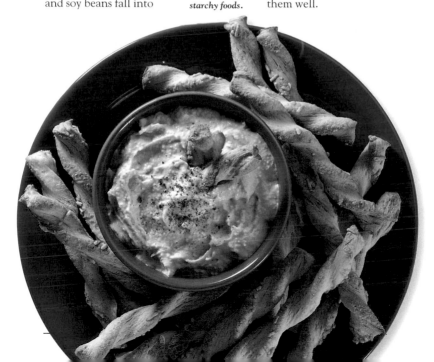

Nuts and seeds

WITH THE EXCEPTION OF *peanuts, all kinds of seeds and nuts can be included as "go-with-anything" foods.*

Nuts are a reasonable source of protein, although not a first class one. They also contain some starch. In addition, they are rich in fat and, although the type of fat is generally of the healthy kind, this high concentration can make nuts difficult to digest. If you like them, but find they disagree with you, crush or grind, and chew them well before swallowing.

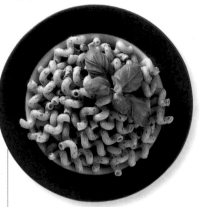

ABOVE **Pesto, a delicious pasta sauce, contains pine nuts.**

Experience shows that most nuts combine in small amounts with either proteins or starches, but that they are digested most easily when mixed only with vegetables or salads.

However, nuts are also a common cause of severe allergic reaction. Peanuts are not nuts, but pulses(see page 38–39).

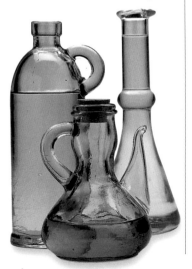

LEFT **Nuts and seeds contain oil which can be used for cooking.**

NUTS	SEEDS
Almonds	Caraway
Brazils	Celery
Cashews	Dill
Chestnuts	Linseeds
Coconuts	Melon
Hazelnuts (Filberts)	Mustard
Macadamia	Poppy
Pecans	Pumpkin
Pine nuts	Sesame
Pistachios	Sunflower
Walnuts	

Although most seeds have a similar nutritional composition to nuts, they do not appear to be difficult to digest. When following a food-combining diet, seeds can be used to "go-with-anything."

Treat sesame seed paste and pesto (which is made with pine nuts) as "go-with-anything" foods.

OILS

The oils that are extracted from nuts and seeds are classed with fats and, as such, combine with starches or proteins.

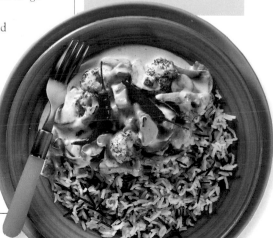

RIGHT **Coconut vegetable curry and fragrant rice.**

Acid/alkaline balance

WHEN FOOD-COMBINING EXPERTS *talk about eating the right ratio of acid-forming to alkaline-forming foods, it can make the whole concept sound complicated. However, the acid/alkali balance is not difficult to understand and is essential to good health.*

Foods are classed, not by how acid or alkaline they are before they are eaten, but by the products they leave in your body after they have been digested, absorbed, and metabolized.

ACID-FORMING FOODS
Protein and starch are turned to acid-forming mineral deposits, including chlorine, phosphorus, and sulfur.

ALKALINE-FORMING FOODS
Vegetables, salads, and fruit are alkaline-forming. They leave residues of magnesium, calcium, iron, and potassium, which help to remove excess acid. Both types of food are essential. The easiest way to achieve a balanced intake of acid- and alkaline-forming foods is

LEFT *Fruit is an alkaline-forming food and helps to rid the body of excess acids.*

to increase the consumption of fresh fruits and vegetables and to ease up on consumption of meat, sugars, and fats.

THE pH SCALE

Acidity and alkalinity are measured on the pH scale. Anything very acid has a low number; anything very alkaline has a high number. Stomach acid has a pH of just above 1; while baking soda has a pH of 12. Water, neither acid nor alkaline, is neutral with a pH of 7. Blood is slightly alkaline, with a pH between 7.35 and 7.45.

Since any deviation in blood pH can cause serious illness, the body has developed a sophisticated mechanism for maintaining equilibrium. However, to help keep this delicate balance, we need to supply plenty of fresh alkaline-forming vegetables and fruits – together with a sensible intake of lean protein and unrefined starches.

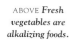

ABOVE *Fresh vegetables are alkalizing foods.*

KEEPING THE BALANCE

To maintain good health, our bodies need to take in a higher level of alkalizing foods than of acid-forming ones. However, to follow the food-combining system successfully, it is not necessary to spend time calculating what percentage of each meal is acid or alkaline.

Alkaline-forming foods

ONE OF THE MOST *interesting findings made by the key food-combining researchers was that people with very acidic blood were more prone to illness and that increasing their intake of alkaline-forming foods led to a number of significant health improvements.*

Whether a food has an alkaline- or acid-forming effect on the body is determined not by how acid or alkaline it is before it's swallowed, but by the type of deposit it leaves behind after it has been metabolized. Proteins are generally acid-forming, but bean curd and yogurt are both alkalizing because they have been through the process of fermentation.

Almost all vegetables, salads, herbs, seeds, pulses, and fresh fruit are alkalizing, but there are

SIMPLY FOLLOW THESE EASY GUIDELINES

● treat all vegetables, salads, and herbs as alkaline-forming

● treat all protein, starches, fats, sugars, and beans as acid-forming

Do not worry about the rest.

some confusing exceptions. Potatoes, classed as starch, are alkaline-forming. Asparagus is believed to be one of the few acid-forming vegetables, and the pulse, or legume, family is listed by some as belonging completely to the acid-forming category.

These minor discrepancies really do not need to be taken into consideration.

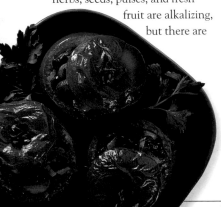

LEFT *A purely alkalizing supper of baked stuffed tomato.*

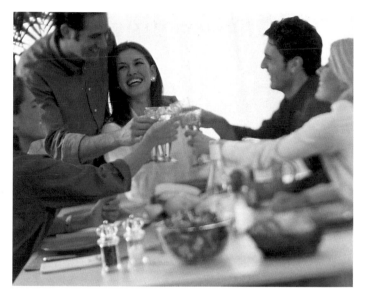

THE BENEFITS OF ALKALIZING FOODS

ABOVE *Relaxation and laughter are alkaline-forming.*

Alkalizing foods act as acid-buffers and are also vital for the structure and repair of every cell in the body. They help to cleanse the system, assisting in the breakdown of wastes and the elimination of toxins. If you are feeling run down or generally out of sorts, a day or two eating just alkalizing salads, vegetables, and fruits can take the strain off an over-worked digestive system.

AN ALKALIZING LIFESTYLE

Rest, sleep, regular exercise, fresh air, laughter, stability, fun, friendship, and love are alkalizing.

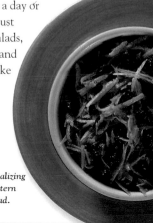

RIGHT *An alkalizing Middle Eastern carrot salad.*

Acid-forming foods

ACID-FORMING FOODS *include most of the proteins (meat, cheese, eggs, fish) and most of the starches (rice, pasta, bread), as well as fats, sugars, and pulses.*

The word "acid" can mean sharp, sour, bitter, acrid. or caustic—terms that apply to personality traits, as well as to food and other substances.

It is thought that eating too many acid-forming foods can make you bad-tempered and irritable and does not encourage good health.

BALANCE IS THE KEY

Proteins and starches are not bad for us. We need to eat food from both the acid-forming and alkaline-forming groups every day, but avoid excess.

LEFT *Asparagus is believed to be one of the few acid-forming vegetables.*

SYMPTOMS OF AN OVER-ACID SYSTEM INCLUDE

- Sluggishness in the morning
- Lethargy after lunch
- Headaches
- Gray pallor
- Oily or dull hair
- Unpleasant body smells
- Sour taste in the mouth
- Bad breath
- Indigestion
- Constipation

Acid saturation is easy to reach if you have a fondness for sweet or fatty foods—pastries, pizzas, burgers, cheese, and so on.

It isn't only an ill-balanced diet that can make the system over-acid. Excess alcohol, smoking, stress, lack of sleep, lack of regular exercise, hyperventilation (fast, shallow breathing), anger, anxiety, envy,

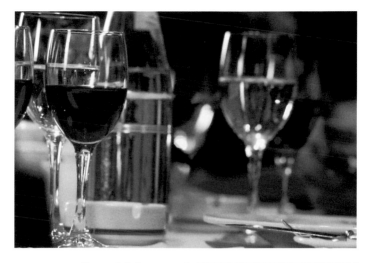

ABOVE *Excess alcohol is acid-forming.*

irritability, panic, fear, and worry are all acid-forming.

We need to include good-quality proteins and starches in our diet every day.

BELOW *Do not overload your body with too many starchy foods, such as pasta. Balance it with vegetable sauces.*

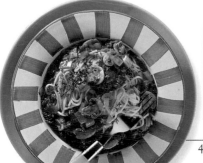

SIMPLE WAYS TO ACHIEVE A BALANCE

● Increase your intake of salad and vegetable produce

●
Include a generous selection of vegetables or salad with every lunch and supper

TOMATOES

CARROTS

● Eat at least two pieces of fresh fruit each day, either between meals or before a main meal.

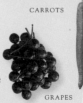

GRAPES

Daily planning

IT IS USUALLY *quite simple to modify your normal eating habits in order to meet the food-combining guidelines.*

Ideally, aim to eat one protein meal with vegetables or salad, one starch meal with vegetables or salad, and one vegetable or fruit only meal.

Modify this to fit in with your daily routine, but maintain a balance throughout the week. For example, one protein and two starch meals, two vegetable and one protein or two protein and one starch meals, over three days.

Include vegetables and salads with as many meals as possible and avoid eating three protein meals or starch meals in a row.

ADAPT YOUR DIET

To plan a food-combined meal imagine what you would ordinarily have eaten, then adapt it to meet the food-combining requirements. For example, if you would have cooked a fish dish with rice and salad, turn it into a protein-based meal by forgetting the rice and choosing a larger portion of fish and salad. To make a starch-based meal, forget the fish, but add other ingredients to the rice, such as beans and vegetables.

MEALTIMES

It is better to leave three to four hours between a protein and starch meal. However, if food is consumed at normal mealtimes, this gap occurs automatically.

DESSERTS

Avoid eating a starch dessert after a protein supper or a protein-based dessert after a starchy meal. It is easier on the digestion – and healthier.

LEFT *Eat fish with salad (rather than potatoes) as a protein meal.*

SUGGESTED DAILY MEAL PLAN

Breakfast 7am

Starch

Brown bread and honey

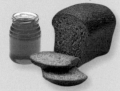

Snack 11am

Fruit

Apple

Lunch 1pm

Starch

Vegetable soup and bread

Dinner 7pm

Protein

Salmon steak and ratatouille

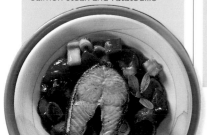

SUGGESTED DAILY MEAL PLAN

Breakfast 7am

Protein

Ham and scrambled eggs

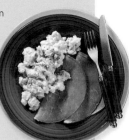

Snack 11am

Fruit

Kiwi fruit

Lunch 1pm

Protein

Shrimp salad

Dinner 7pm

Starch

Pasta and vegetables

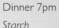

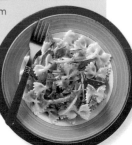

Starch-based meals

AS YOU GET MORE USED TO *the food-combining diet, it will become easier to choose starch-based meals. The following meal suggestions will help you to get started with a food-combining regime. Modify them to suit your own tastes.*

BREAKFASTS

Oatmeal porridge—make it with water and serve with cold-pressed honey and cream.

Crusty wholegrain or soda bread and honey—use a close-textured bread (not processed) and cold-pressed, raw honey.

Mushrooms on toast—sauté the mushrooms in olive oil and serve on wholegrain toast.

Muesli with almond milk—use any good quality oat-based cereal and make almond milk by blending a dozen blanched almonds with half a cup of water.

ABOVE *Sautéed mushrooms on wholegrain toast.*

Rice cakes and sugar-free preserve—these also make a good snack between meals.

SNACKS AND SUPPERS

Baked potato—vary the theme by adding hummus, chopped broiled mushrooms,

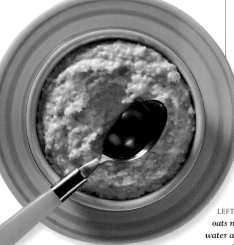

LEFT *Porridge oats made with water and served with honey.*

pesto, mayonnaise, baked beans, or coleslaw and serve with salad or vegetables.

Baked beans on toast—a filling starch snack on its own.

Tomato and lettuce sandwich—delicious served with corn chips.

Pasta salad—use cooked pasta shells or twists, tossed in dressing or mayonnaise, and served with a salad. Serve hot in winter.

Potato and onion salad—use either new or maincrop potatoes, scrub them, leaving on the skins, and cook in salted water. Drain, cut into cubes, and fry with a

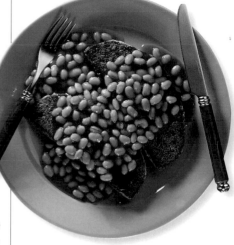

ABOVE *Baked beans on toast is a wholesome, starchy supper*

chopped onion in olive oil. Serve with salad and brown bread.

Baguette or ciabatta—dunked in olive oil and spread with hummus.

Brown rice and beans – use any kind of pulse except soy. Add sliced green beans, fresh peas, fried mushrooms, and onions for extra quantity, texture, and flavor.

LEFT *Serve a hot baked potato with coleslaw and salad for a filling lunch.*

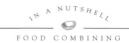
Protein-based meals

PROTEIN IS ESSENTIAL FOR THE BODY *to function. It plays an important role in the repair and growth of cells and should make up about 15 per cent of your food intake. Here are some tasty ways to include protein in your daily diet.*

BREAKFASTS

Strained yogurt with chopped banana and honey —choose sheep's milk yogurt, if possible, and on colder mornings slice the bananas lengthwise and broil them quickly first.
Scrambled eggs—use two eggs and add lean ham, flaked salmon, or grated cheese.

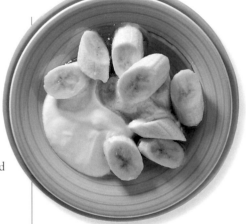

ABOVE *Banana and yogurt—a quick, easy protein breakfast.*

Lean bacon slices with broiled tomatoes—broil both the bacon and tomatoes.
Vegetarian sausage with mushrooms and tomatoes–all these can be broiled too.

LEFT *A weekend protein treat—bacon and tomatoes.*

Hunza apricots with yogurt—
soak the apricots in water
overnight. Hunza apricots are
available from health stores
and some delicatessens.

SNACKS AND SUPPERS

Omelet—use two eggs
and fill with grated
cheese, chopped spinach,
or fried onion.

Cheese salad – try using
goats or sheeps cheese and
break into a large bowl of salad.
Include lettuce, tomato, fresh

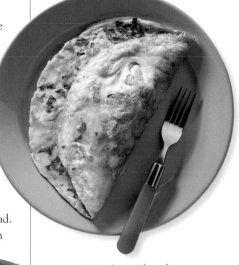

ABOVE *A spinach omelet
is a quick,
tasty evening meal.*

herbs, grated
zucchini, grated
carrot, chopped
celery, and sliced
bell pepper.
**Salmon, tuna, or
sardine salad—**
make this in the
same way as cheese
salad, but swap the
cheese for fish.

LEFT *What could
be simpler than a
cheese salad?*

Fruits, vegetables, and salads

TRY TO INCLUDE AS MANY VARIETIES *of fruit and vegetables in your diet as possible. Fruit is an excellent way to start the day and a snack can mean a healthy bowl of soup.*

BREAKFASTS

Fresh fruit salad—make a generous-sized fresh fruit salad using at least three pieces of fruit. Choose from kiwis, pears, peaches, nectarines, grapes, mandarins, clementines, pineapples, and mangoes.

Fresh fruit drink—a refreshing alternative to fruit salad is to blend three fruits into juice.

Fruit compote — dried fruit, soaked

LEFT **Nothing beats the taste of freshly squeezed orange.**

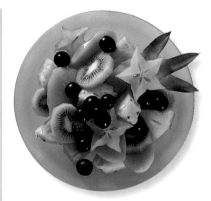

ABOVE **A fruit salad will give you energy for the day ahead.**

overnight, makes a sweet and satisfying breakfast dish. Figs, yellow apricots, Hunza apricots, seedless raisins, and dried bananas are all good choices.

Fruit and vegetable drink—carrot, raw beet, apple, and grapes make an unusual, sweet, and extremely healthy breakfast juice.

SNACKS AND SUPPERS

Vegetable soup—cook a variety of vegetables until they are tender and blend them into soup. Add sea salt, black pepper, and herbs for extra flavor. Serve with crusty bread or rye crackers for a starch meal; add grated cheese or a handful of cooked shrimp for a protein meal.

Vegetable compote—on chillier days, a variety of cooked vegetables can make a filling lunch. Choose broccoli, carrot, rutabaga or zucchini.

Tomato salad with black olives and balsamic dressing—peel and slice two or three tomatoes, garnish with black olives, and

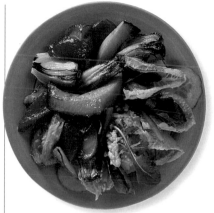

ABOVE *Roast vegetables and serve with salad greens.*

sprinkle with a simple dressing made with balsamic vinegar and extra virgin olive oil.

Corn cobs`—serve with melted butter.

Roasted vegetables—sliced eggplant, bell peppers, tomatoes, zucchini, and baby corn, lightly salted, drizzled with olive oil, and cooked under the broiler or on the barbecue. Serve with salad.

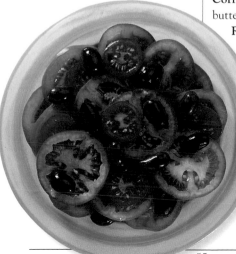

LEFT *This delicately flavored tomato and olive salad can be served with any meal.*

Exceptions to the rule

ALTHOUGH THE PRINCIPLES OF FOOD COMBINING *are very simple, it is not always easy to work out how particular foods should be classified.*

Cream, which is made from milk, is a "go-with-anything" food, while milk is classed as a protein. The reason is the quantity of fat. Ordinary pasteurized whole milk has a fat content of around ½ ounce per ⅔ cup; but the same amount of double cream has 4¼ ounces of fat. However, we use far less cream than milk, and although the protein content is about the same, food-combining experience has shown that small quantities of cream are compatible with protein or starch. Milk, on the other hand, does not mix happily with starchy foods.

ABOVE **Fruit salad accompanied by "go-with-anything" cream.**

PASTA— PROTEIN OR STARCH?

Pasta has an apparent dual composition —it is primarily a starch, but some pastas are made with egg, a protein. In fact, the nutritional make-up of pasta varies very little whether it contains egg

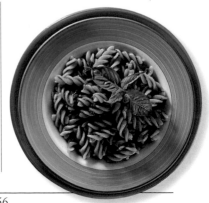

RIGHT **Fusilli with tomato and garlic is a starch meal.**

or not. For the purposes of food combining, all plain pasta is a starchy food and, therefore, combines well with any of the "go-with-anything" foods.

However, pasta served with sauces or fillings made from meat or cheese is a mix of concentrated starch and protein and, as such, is best kept for non-combining days.

SUGARY FOODS

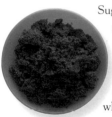

Sugar plays a far greater role in our diet today than it used to and is, in fact, a refined carbohydrate, which means that it fits into the starch category.

ABOVE **Sugar counts as a starch.**

SAUCES AND GRAVIES

Sauces and gravies can be confusing. Any sauce that is made with flour (starch) and milk (protein) is providing an unacceptable combination, even though the amounts

per serving are relatively small.

Gravy, made with flour, would not work well with a protein meal, as far as food combining is concerned. However, occasional sauces and gravies added to either protein or starch meals do not appear to disturb digestion to any great extent.

ABOVE **Gravy can be served with meat occasionally.**

DESSERTS

Sweet desserts will interfere with stomach acid if eaten after a protein meal. Try to keep sweet foods to a minimum—eat them on their own or after a starch meal, rather than a protein one.

ABOVE **Try not to eat a sweet dessert after a protein meal, such as stir fried bean curd.**

Further reading

HOW TO DINE LIKE THE DEVIL AND FEEL LIKE A SAINT, *Luc DeSchepper* (Full of Life Publishing, 1993)

FOODS COMBINING DIET, *Kathryn Marsden* (Thorsons, 1993)

FOOD COMBINING MEAL PLANS, *Kathryn Marsden* (Thorsons, 1994)

EATING ALIVE, *Dr. Jonn Matsen* (Crompton Books 1991)

BETTER HEALTH THROUGH NATURAL HEALING, *Ross Trattler* (Thorsons, 1987)

THE WRIGHT DIET, *Celia Wright* (Green Library, 1991)

FOOD COMBINING IN THIRTY DAYS, *Kathryn Marsden* (Thorsons, 1994)

FOOD AND HEALING, *Annemarie Colbin* (Ballantine Books, 1986)

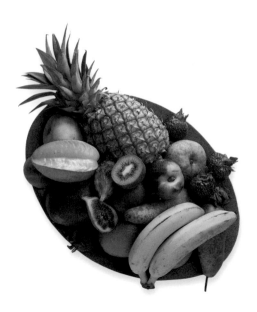

Useful addresses

The Vegetarian Society
Parkdale
Durham Rd
Altrincham
Cheshire WA14 4QG,
England

**The Vegetarian Union of
North America**
PO Box 9710
Washington DC20016
USA

**The Australian
Vegetarian Society**
PO Box 65
2021, Paddington
Australia

The Soil Association
86, Colston St
Bristol BS1 5BB
England

Farm Verified Organic
RR 1
Box 40A USA
Medina ND 58467
USA

**National Association for
Sustainable Agriculture**
PO Box 768
AUS-Sterling
SA5152
Australia

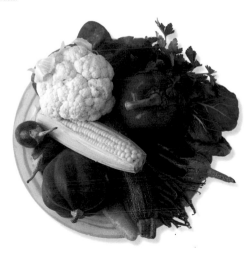